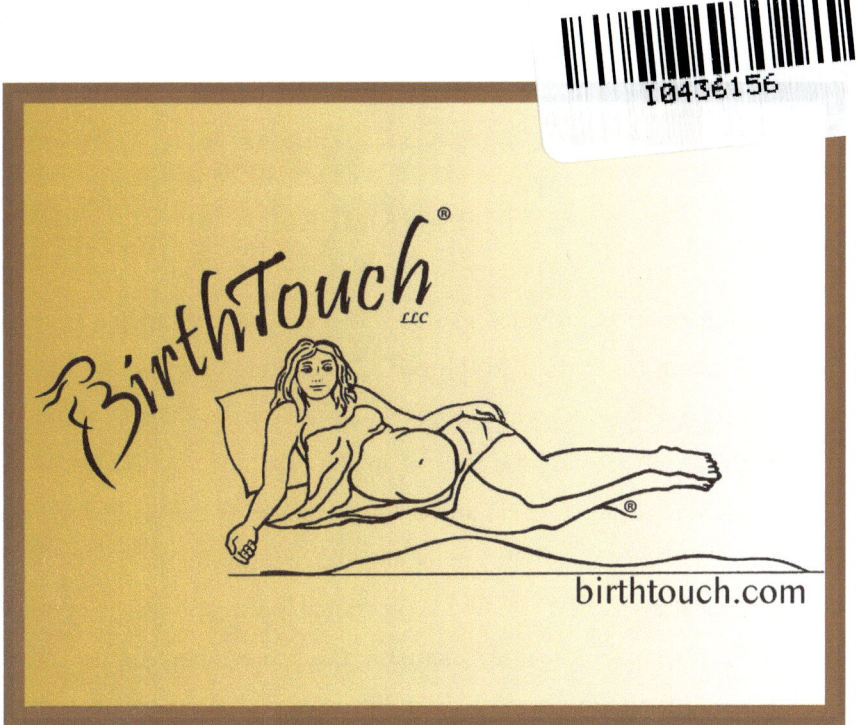

DISCLAIMER

The information provided in this site is not medical advice. Birth-Touch® Healing for Parents in the NICU is intended for use by healthy adults to cope with stress while in hospital waiting rooms and at home.

BirthTouch® Healing for Parents in the NICU is not a diagnosis or treatment and is not intended in any way to diagnose or treat an individual. Nothing in this document is meant to suggest, circumvent, replace, or contradict medical advice and care by a professional health care provider, other medical professional or licensed mental health professional. Consult with your professional health-care provider, other medical professional or licensed mental health professional before using BirthTouch® Healing for Parents in the NICU. The use of the information provided by BirthTouch® Healing for Parents in the NICU is at the sole risk of the user. BirthTouch® Healing for Parents in the NICU, on behalf of itself, its author and publisher, disclaim all conditions, express or implied, arising by law or otherwise, with respect to the use of the information contained herein and further disclaim any liability for loss or damages, personal or otherwise resulting from the information or use of information contained in this publication and shall not be liable to the user or any third party for any damages, special, punitive, incidental, indirect, consequential or otherwise.

ACKNOWLEDGMENTS

Thanks to my many teachers and friends who have shared with me shiatsu, acupressure, and Reiki, clinical psychology, life, and love!

Special shout out to my wonderful family for their love and support, many thanks Bill and Will!

Illustration by Noreen Morelli
Cover Design: Will Kenly

Photography: David Ammirata www.theammiratas.com
Model: Britni Morley
Hair by Keri Ann
Cover Photography: Istock/YanC
Copyright 2012 by Kathy Morelli
Published by BirthTouch®, LLC

ISBN-13: 9781475257243

ISBN-10: 1475257244

BIRTHTOUCH®
HEALING FOR PARENTS IN THE NICU

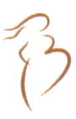

Table of Contents

FOREWORD

by Leslie Butterfield, Ph.D.

Research tells us that gentle touch heals, and that couples who "turn toward" one another enjoy more satisfactory and enduring marriages. Couples with a baby in the NICU undergo tremendous physical and emotional stress, often tinged with loneliness, anxiety and grief.

BirthTouch® Healing for Parents in the NICU provides a simple and straightforward way for couples to provide one another with physical and emotional support - even if their coping styles differ and their grieving patterns are uniquely individual or their stress responses aren't alike at all.

The lovely pairing of her HEALING WORDS with the various SHIATSU TECHNIQUES ensures the positivity gained through practicing therapeutic touch will remain in the body memory as each parent (or family member) moves through the frequent ups and downs that accompany NICU stays.

The illustrations are an excellent visual guide, while the healing words offer a verbal pathway to mutual caring. Take the pocket guide with you – you can use these techniques at the hospital or at home, and you can share them with others.

Leslie Butterfield, Ph.D. is a clinical psychologist specializing in perinatal and reproductive health concerns. She has an active clinical practice and teaches at the Seattle Midwifery School and the Department of Midwifery at Bastyr Naturopathic University. She is the Chairwoman of Postpartum Support International for Washington State and is the Vice President of Prevention and Treatment of Traumatic Childbirth. Dr. Butterfield is married and is the mother of two teenage boys.

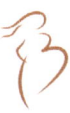

Introduction

BirthTouch® Seated Shiatsu is a simple, safe shiatsu seated routine to be used for healing and self-care by couples experiencing distress in the NICU. It is designed to help women and their families create a holding environment of safety during the crisis of experiencing a premature birth.

In Each Step of BirthTouch®
Seated Shiatsu, are Words That Heal.

It is my hope that when you feel angry with the world and each other about what has happened, safe touch and self-care and understanding can be a small way to help you turn towards each other rather than away.

This short handbook is dedicated to support staff and couples looking for a simple way to provide comfort to each other. Simple touch helps soothe feelings of anxiety. It is a low-cost self-help way to soothe raw emotional wounds.

Touch is a way to help couples and families restore intimacy and trust, to reduce their anger towards the world and each other, a way to purposefully and ritualistically contain the pain and to reconnect through the distress.

Anxiety and body tension can really build in an emergency situation.

Simple touch and simple safe words invoke the relaxation response and promote feelings of safety and bonding.

I do hope you find the material useful.

If you are feeling very anxious, depressed, and/or panicky, you must seek professional help. Please see your primary care physician or a licensed mental health professional for an assessment. BirthTouch® is to be used as self-help, complementary care.

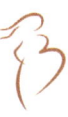

Words That Heal

We are both hurt and angry, let's vow not to take it out on each other.

It's not your fault.

We are both doing the best we can.

Let's lean on each other.

We have life skills, we can use them together now.

Together, we'll make it.

Let's pray together.

Our friends and family will help us, we have to ask.

Actions That Heal

Refrain from the blame game.

Keep your heart soft and turn towards your partner.

Realize anger is normal, taking it out on your partner is unfair and hurts. This behavior can permanently damage the relationship.

Vent to someone who understands that you are hurt, angry and need a release for normal feelings, not exclusively to your partner.

Allow yourself to sometimes forget the pain and even laugh. This is a normal emotional flow, and is a protective device, allowing you some respite from intense emotion.

Practice lovingkindness towards oneself and others.

Give yourself a break from the pain by asking it to take a rest. You can give your pain a name, and a persona, too, and ask it to go to sleep, so you can have some respite. For example, imagine your pain to be a cat named Harry. Ask Harry to go to sleep on his bed in the corner for now while you have a rest.

Connect with your wider faith, whatever that means to you, such as Christianity, Judaism, Native American.

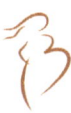

Self-Care Heals

Self-care is important in the best of times, yet even more so during stressful times. You may be so overwhelmed that taking care of yourself seems irrelevant. Mindbody practices are inexpensive self-care practices that can be used at any time for anxiety reduction. You know that your entire being will suffer on several different levels if you do not take care of your self.

As hard as it sounds, you need to value yourself during this crisis. Valuing yourself through a crisis can be as simple as eating as well as possible, sleeping or at least, resting, and managing your emotional swings. Be kind to yourself during this painful time.

Square Breathing

This is easy to practice. When you feel yourself tightening up, take a deep breath and then scan your body, and let yourself relax from the scalp down to your toes.

* Breath in for a count of three, hold it for a three, breathe out for three, and hold there for three.

Autogenic Relaxation

This is simply a full body relaxation developed by Johannes Heinrich Schultz in 1932.

It is simply imagining the parts of your body getting heavy and warm, little by little.

Take an easy, slow breath. Think:

My body easily breathes itself.

My neck is comfortably warm and heavy.

My arms are comfortably heavy & warm.

My heartbeat is strong and steady.

My stomach feels comfortably heavy & warm

My body breathes itself.

My legs are comfortably heavy & warm.

My heartbeat is strong and steady.

My body is relaxed.

Circle of Peace Meditation

Create your Circle of Peace by just closing your eyes, taking three deep slow breaths and imagining a beautiful circle of fire protecting you. You are completely safe inside this circle. You can imagine a spiritual being drawing this circle of fire around you, perhaps an angel, or the Archangel Michael, whomever you trust. It can be any color you wish, blue, green, yellow....Take some time to create it... You can make it very big or just let it hug your body. Just make sure it is all positive for you. You can get strength from a team of helpers (real-life or imaginary) bringing you support. Add their goodwill to your spiritual being. Take a deep breath and sigh, and let your Circle of Peace become a place you can always go to if you need to. If there is negativity around you, you can stop it with your Circle of Peace. Take a deep breath and relax.

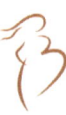

BirthTouch® Healing for Parents in the NICU

BirthTouch® in the NICU: Seated Shiatsu

Touch is a way to help couples and families restore intimacy and trust, to reduce their anger towards the world and each other, a way to purposefully and ritualistically contain the pain and to reconnect through the distress.

I invite you to use simple touch to invoke the relaxation response and promote feelings of safety and bonding and to use the Words that Heal to turn towards each other

BirthTouch® Seated Shiatsu Step by Step instructions follow.

BirthTouch® Step-by-Step Seated Shiatsu Routine

Step One. Create your loving intention and emotional connection.

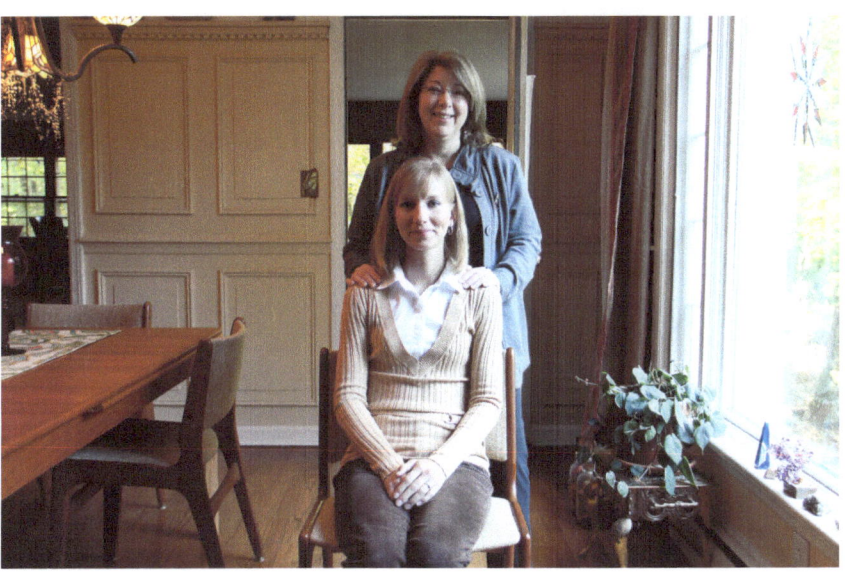

Begin by positioning your partner in a chair. Stand behind her. Connect with her emotionally and energetically by resting your hands on her shoulders. Center yourself with loving intention by taking a few easy breaths.

Words that Heal: We are both hurt and angry, let's vow not to take it out on each other.

Step Two. Relaxing scalp circles.

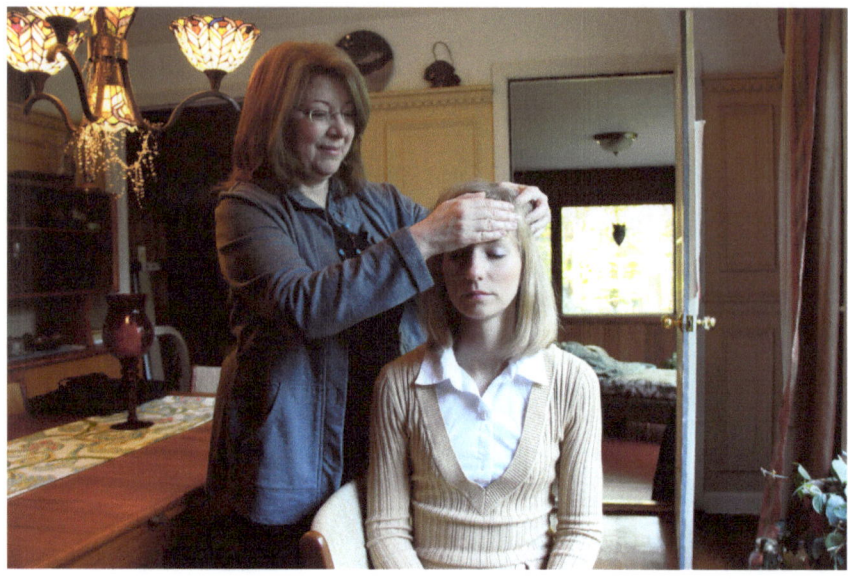

Support your partner's head by placing your hand on her forehead. With your free hand, help her relax by massaging the scalp with your fingers. The scalp as many nerve endings, thus many people find this relaxing.

Words that Heal: Let's open to our healing powers.

Step Three. Circles along the base of the head to relax both head & neck.

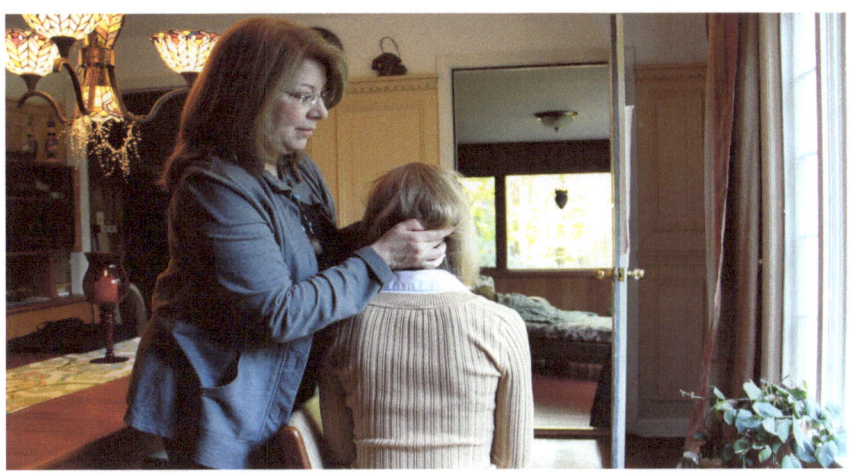

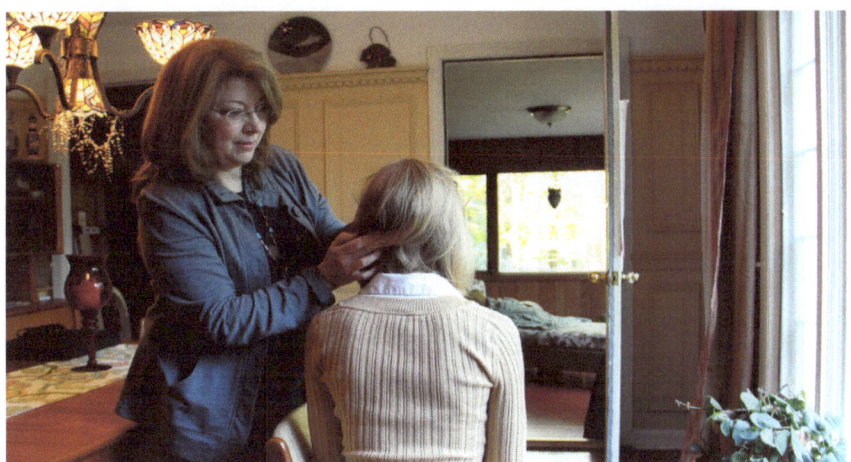

Still supporting your partner's head with your hand on her forehead, use your fingers to make small circles along the base of the skull, or the occipital ridge. Start from the center of the skull and work outward to the ear. Do this on both sides. This will help loosen both head and neck muscles.

Words that Heal: It's not your fault.

Step Four. Relieve neck tension.

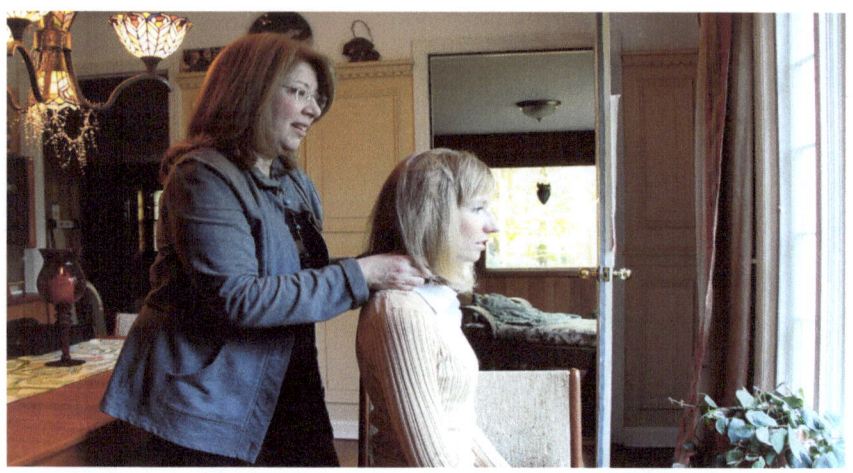

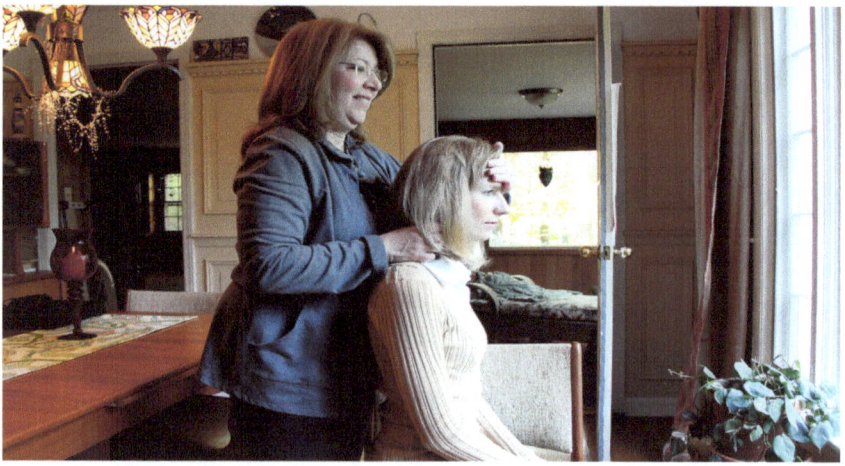

Next, relax your partner's neck by stroking the back of her neck on each side of the cervical spine. Stroke three times on each side, using a caring, rhythmic touch. You can still support her head with your free hand on her forehead.

Words that Heal: We are both doing the best we can.

Step Five. Warm up the shoulder and arm muscles.

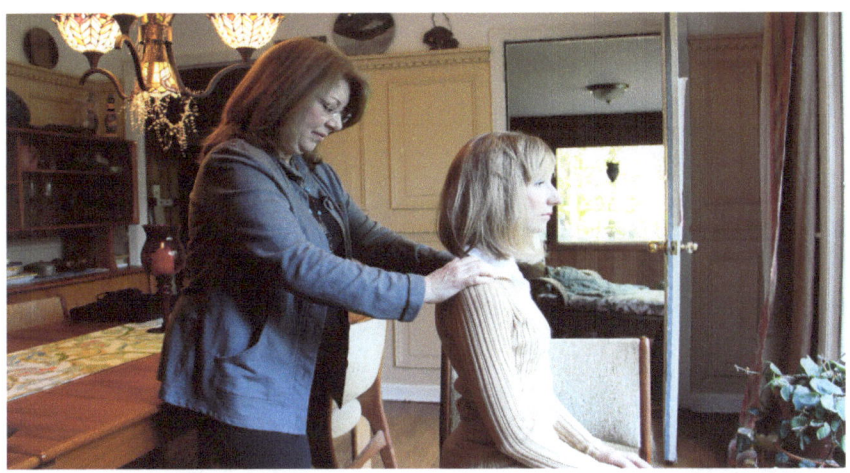

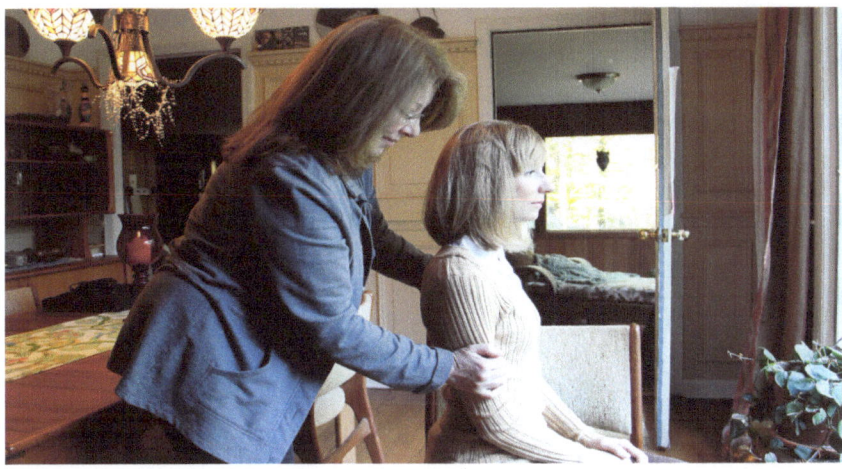

Now warm up and relax your partner's shoulders by using your hands to squeeze out from the neck to the end of the shoulders three times. The, move down to your partner's arms and squeeze down the arms three times, starting from the shoulders to the elbow. This work prepares the body for the next move.

Words that Heal: Let's lean on each other.

Step Six. Rotate the shoulders to move the stress out!

*** Skip this step if your partner has shoulder problems. ***

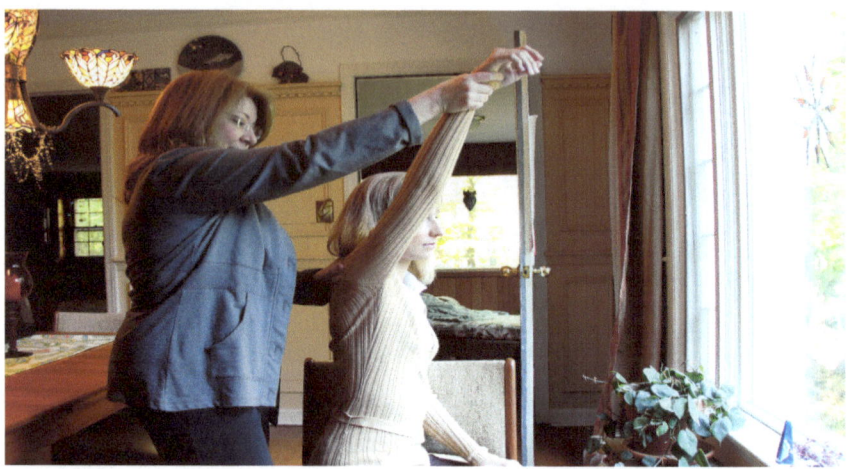

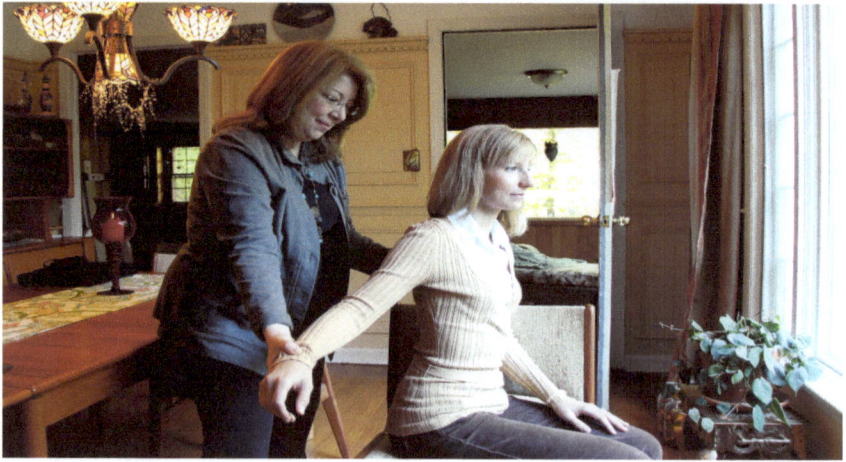

Once the shoulder area has been loosened up a bit by squeezing the neck and arms, you can very carefully rotate your partner's arm. Use one hand as an anchor on her shoulder, hold above her wrist with your other hand, and very slowly and carefully rotate her arm. Strive to understand her range of motion, to not try to rotate beyond the natural range of motion.

Step easily forward and backward yourself to create and follow the motion.

Words that Heal: We have life skills, we can use them together now.

Step Seven. For comfort, reduce the tightness in the large back muscles.

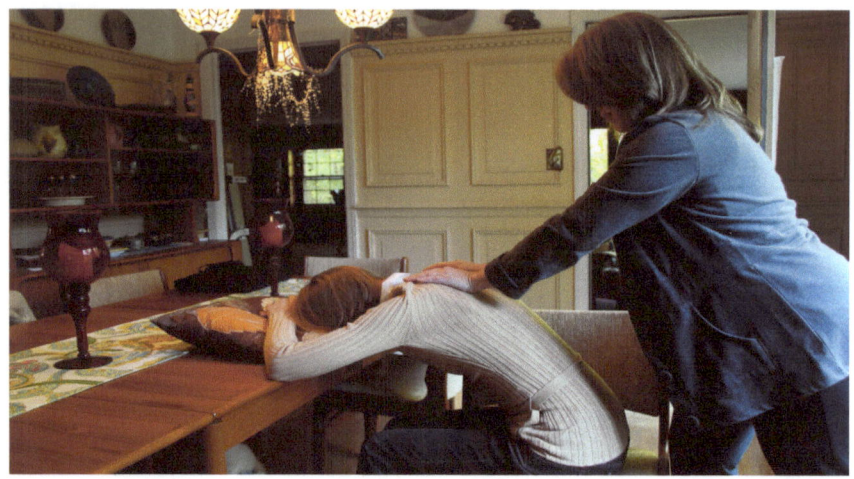

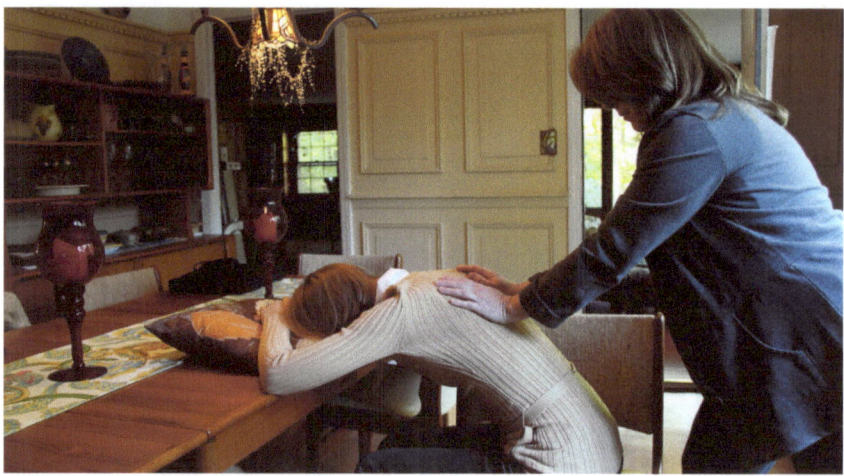

Help her relax her back. Have your partner rest her head on a pillow on a table. To protect your own back, use both your hands, lean in from your center, and work with one foot slightly behind the other. Work from the top of her back down to the base of her back, press with the heels of your hands, leaning in with your body weight, rather than using your strength. Avoid the spine, and press in the channel on either side of the spine. Do this three times.

Words that Heal: Together, we'll make it.

Step Eight. Move the stress out of the sacral and hip area.

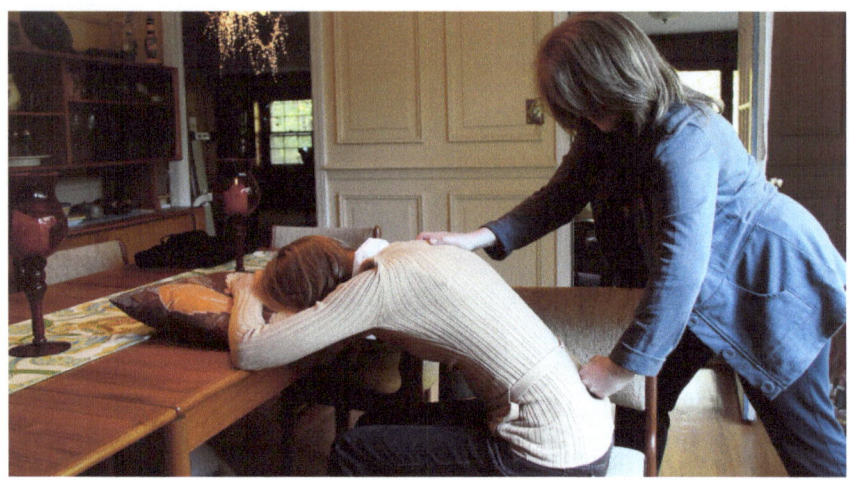

You can move a lot of stress out of the sacral and hip areas by using your fists on the big muscular areas, avoiding the bony areas. Rub the area using one or both of your fists. To protect your own back, place one foot slightly in front of the other, and use your body weight to press in with your fist.

Words that Heal: Let's pray together.

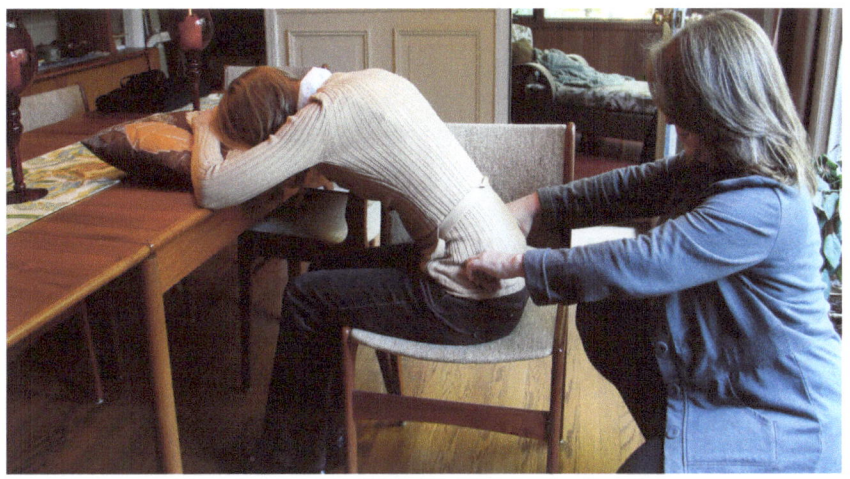

Hip release. Squat down to protect your own back. Press into the hip areas, avoiding the bony areas, with your hands on either side of your partners hips.

Step 9. Release the large muscles of the thighs. .

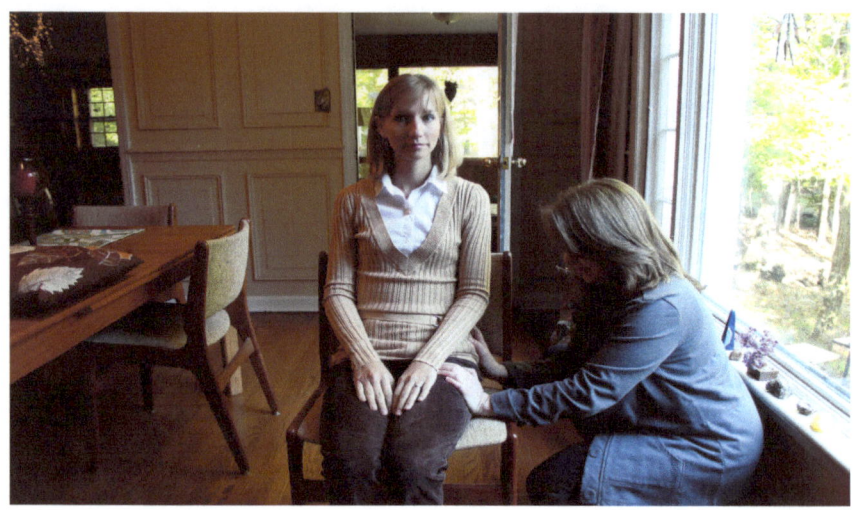

Squatting down, press the side of the thigh from the hip down to the knee three times.

Words that Heal: our friends and family will help us, we have to ask

Conclusion

Staying physically and mentally healthy will help you cope with the challenge of being a parent of a baby in the NICU, help support each other as partners. Simple self-care methods such as slow breathing, conscious relaxation of muscle tension, taking short walks, easy stretches, watching your sugar and caffeine intake and looking for whole food choices are basic ways to take care of your body and emotional health.

About the Author

Kathy Morelli, Director of BirthTouch® LLC is an author, speaker and Licensed Professional Counselor. Her private practice is in Wayne, NJ and centers on marriage and family counseling with a special interest in the emotions of pregnancy, birth, postpartum, and trauma.

She offers consultation sessions via Skype. She can be reached via Skype at KathyNJLPC and her websites: Birthtouch.com, Kathy Morelli.com and Mental Health Support Online.Com

She has been married for 22 years and has a teenage son. She volunteers for Postpartum Support International's warmline and is the creator and co-moderator of #MHON, a weekly Twitter chat provided as a public health service, featuring licensed mental health professionals disseminating information on their expertise.